# Postpartum Depression

## A Parent's Guide To Postpartum Depression

# Published By Shaharm Publications

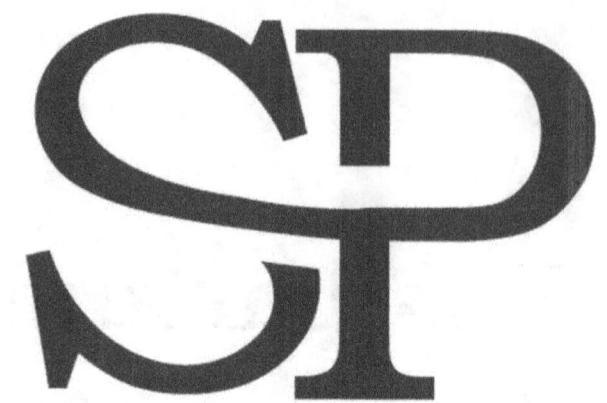

For a full list of books by Shaharm Publications, please go to:

http://www.shaharmpublications.com

# TABLE OF CONTENTS

# INTRODUCTION

After giving birth, many moms find that they are not overcome with the joy that they expected to feel after delivering their child. While this may seem like a bad way to begin your journey into motherhood, it is actually a common issue. Feelings of depression can creep in and overshadow any positive feelings connected to the arrival of the baby. You may have the desire to be happy and enjoy the new addition to your family, but this is much easier to say than it is to realize.

Many women experience a depressed mood after delivering a child.

There have been numerous works that have fictionalized "baby blues," and trivialize the issue, but this is not the case at all. Unfortunately, some people are so depressed after having a child that they are at risk to harm to themselves and/or the baby. This cannot be prevented if people are not willing to address this as a genuine issue and seek the proper assistance.

Reaching out for help is sometimes seen as letting the world know that you are weak, or that you are not strong enough to handle life as well as everyone else can. Honestly, people who are able to spot the problem and look for solutions are very strong. Yes, they may have a difficult time handling their emotions right now, but they realize that something is wrong and they ask for help; that is something that should be commended.

This is not a problem that plagues every woman that gives birth. There are even some people who refuse to believe that this is a real issue. They think that it is as simple as willing yourself to think positively. Others are under the false impression that you can snap your fingers, love your baby and use that as motivation to feel better. If it were that simple, there wouldn't be mothers out there who feel as if they are sinking into the blues.

Years ago it used to be a stigma to find a therapeutic solution for problems. Many people struggled to deal with emotional issues on their own, and those who sought help did so under a thick cloud of secrecy. If you are having dealing with postpartum depression, you need to understand that you are not alone. Between 10 and 15 percent of new moms experience this problem.

There is no magical formula recipe that makes up a woman who suffers from postpartum depression (also known as postnatal depression). Yes, there are some risk factors that may make some people more susceptible, but this is not something that can be positively predicted. Women of all different ages, cultures, races and socioeconomic backgrounds have suffered; many have done so in silence.

It is time to step out from the shadows and address this issue. As long as it is treated as if it is some dreadful disease, people will continue to hide it and they will not get the help that they so desperately need. The following guide will discuss this issue in depth. You will learn everything about it, including how to spot the signs, where to go for help and different treatment options. This has to be handled for the sake of you, your children and your emotional well being.

# RECOGNIZING THE SIGNS

Everyone who feels a little down in the dumps after having a baby does not have postnatal depression. There are some clear signs that the issue is more serious than simply having a bad day. Here are some of the signals that you should be on the lookout for. If you notice one or more of them, you should seek help to ensure the problems are not allowed to fester.

## Loss Of Appetite

If you notice that you are not eating as much as normal, this is one of the more common signs of postnatal depression. This is not something that you should take lightly, especially if you are breastfeeding your child. You cannot expect to keep them in the best of health if you are not nourishing your body as well as possible. Not feeling hungry every once in a while is normal, but you should be concerned if this is an ongoing thing.

## Extreme Fatigue

It can be pretty difficult to get yourself on a regular sleep schedule after the baby comes, but you should have adjusted within the first few weeks. If you notice that you are extremely tired all of the time, even when you have slept the proper number of hours the night before, this may be cause for concern.

Inability To Bond With The Baby

You are a new mom and this may require some getting used to, but if you feel no type of bond with your child that is a huge warning sign. Parenthood is an emotionally charged time rife with feelings of love and attachment. Having a lack of emotions toward your baby is something that needs to be addressed as soon as possible. You do not want it to have a negative effect on the growth and development of your child.

## Withdrawing

Having time alone is completely normal, but you should not feel like you need to be cut off from the world. If you are one of those people who are usually surrounded by others, yet all you are consumed with right now is the thought of being alone, that is a serious warning sign. Solitary time is something that everyone craves and values, yet this should not be the new standard for you.

## Increased Irritability

Whether they want to admit it or not, everyone out there has people and things that get on their nerves. This can cause then to feel frustrated and rather irritable. In the case of many people who have experienced postpartum depression, there is no blatant reason for them to feel this sense of irritation. In fact, they can become increasingly irritated as the day progresses; even while there is nothing going on.

## Insomnia

Waking up at all hours of the night to check on the baby can be difficult, and it sometimes leads to sleeping trouble. Even so, if you notice that you are unable to sleep for extended periods of time, you should be concerned and take note. Part of being a great mom is being well rested and ready to care for your child. Being awake for days on end is a serious problem that needs to be addressed.

## Thoughts Of Harming Yourself Or The Baby

Unfortunately, there are some mothers who are so overwhelmed by the emotions they are experiencing that they have given thought to hurting themselves or their baby. If you have been thinking that life would be better without one or both of you, it is important for you to seek help as soon as you can before it is far too late.

Those are many of the signs of postnatal depression. If you have experienced one or more of these since you have given birth, you should be concerned. While it may turn out that the symptoms are not quite as serious as you had previously thought, it is best to err on the side of caution. You need to get to a doctor so you can get the proper diagnosis.

# GETTING A PROPER DIAGNOSIS

Instead of sitting around and wondering if the problems you have experienced are related to postnatal depression, you should focus on getting a diagnosis. Perhaps you have simply been having a case of the baby blues, but you will never know unless you seek the help of a professional. Here are a few tips that will help you along the way.

**Talk To Your Obstetrician/Gynecologist**

You are not the first woman that has experienced these symptoms and you most certainly will not be the last. It is very likely that your doctor has seen this before and they will know exactly what to do. It may be possible for them to speak with you and give you a rudimentary diagnosis, but the best thing to do would be to ask them for a referral. They can lead you to a provider that may be more skilled at helping you with this particular problem.

**Checking Your Thyroid**

Before signing on the dotted line and giving you a referral to a mental health provider, your doctor may want to check your thyroid. There are several postpartum depression symptoms that are the same as the signs of thyroid problems, including problems with appetite and feelings if extreme fatigue. This is not a lengthy procedure. You will only need to agree to a blood test in order to find out if this is the root of your issues.

**Submitting To A Questionnaire**

When you arrive at your doctor's office and let them know what you have been experiencing lately, they may ask you to fill out a few forms so they can get a better idea of what you are going through. These questions will ask you about how intense your feelings are and how often you experience them. It is also likely to include questions about the dates when you first started to feel this way. Being truthful on these forms is the only way that you will get the proper help.

**Get A Second Opinion**

As with any serious diagnosis you have ever received, it is always best to get a second opinion. You do not want to start treating a serious condition only to realize that your issue is temporary blues. You also do not want to take a chance that you actually have a more serious problem, namely postpartum psychosis, and the treatment you receive is not enough to handle the problem.

**Be Open To Change**

You may wonder what this has to do with getting a diagnosis, but it is fairly simple: Getting a diagnosis is pretty useless if you do not plan to take any steps to correct the problem. There are many people who walk into the doctor's office and cry for help, yet they are not receptive when it comes to the treatment options available to them. A doctor can only help you if this is something that you truly want.

In order to begin treating someone for postpartum depression, it is important that this is determined to be the cause of the problems they have been having. After reading this, you should be more than ready to go and find out if this is what has been plaguing you. This is an important step in the process and it can be quite frightening, but it is necessary if you are hoping for things to take a positive turn in the future.

# EXPLORING MEDICAL TREATMENTS

There are several medical treatments available for people who have postpartum. Other options exist as well, and they will be discussed in the next couple of sections. People who have more severe symptoms are generally given medical treatment options. This is because you will start to have noted improvement right away, as opposed to waiting for the result of months of counseling. If you are unaware of what medical treatments may be available, it would be best to continue reading.

**Hormone Therapy**

Estrogen levels are greatly affected when you give birth to a child. Sometimes this large hormonal change is enough to cause postpartum depression. There is very limited evidence to support the idea that offering women hormone therapy will be a cure-all for their problems, but it is most certainly worth a shot. There are some risks involved with this, which may include:

- Headache

- Nausea

- Retention of fluids

- Weight gain

- Vaginal discharge

There is a chance that you will experience all of these as a result of hormone therapy, but there is also a chance you will not. This is something that should be thoroughly discussed with your doctor.

## Antidepressants

Since this is a form of depression, it is only expected that you can treat this the way you would any other. There are multiple antidepressants on the market and your doctor may want to prescribe one for you. The one they recommend will depend on several factors, so there is no way to tell what you will be offered ahead of time. In order to maximize the benefit of any drugs that are prescribed, you should follow these simple rules:

1. Take Them As Prescribed – There are many people who feel that it is okay to stop taking prescription drugs because they are starting the feel better. The thing about antidepressants is that they are a long-term solution. You will need to take them on an ongoing basis to have the best results.

2. Ask About Interactions – If you are currently taking any type of medication regularly, prescription and non-prescription, let your doctor know right away. You do not want to begin a course of treatment that can cause things to become worse instead of better. Even if the medications you are taking are as harmless as aspirin, but it is a good idea to check anyway.

3. Ask About Breastfeeding – You do not want to put anything in your body that may harm your child, so ask about any antidepressants before you take them. Generally, many women breastfeed and take prescription drugs, but it is a good idea to double-check before it is too late.

Antidepressants are generally offered to people in correlation with counseling. They are often prescribed when it seems like mental health counseling is not having the desired result. One thing is certain: You should only take antidepressants that are prescribed to you. Trying to self-diagnose and treat the problem with ill-gotten drugs can cause grave danger to you and/or your baby.

These are the two medical treatments that are usually offered to women who have been diagnosed with postpartum depression. They are not a mandatory part of treatment, but they should most certainly be considered.

# TIPS FOR GETTING THE MOST FROM COUNSELING

If you have decided to seek mental health counseling as a treatment for postpartum depression, good for you! This is a well-proven way to get the help you need and restore order in your life. One thing you should know is that counseling is not about performing magic. You cannot expect it to work if you are not willing to work with it. Try these tips if you want to have the best possible experience.

## Find Someone You Like

One thing that is true of most people is that they will never feel 100% comfortable sharing with someone they do not like. Even though getting counseling is not about finding a close, personal friend, your counselor is someone that you will need to confide in and share things with you may not feel are worth sharing with others. With that being said, go for a consultation with several counselors before selecting one. That is the best way to ensure you will be making the right choice.

## Learn Now To Listen

While you may have the desire to go into your counseling sessions, vent and go home, it is important that you learn to listen to your counselor. After listening to what you have to say, they should be ready to offer you sound feedback. If you are not willing to be receptive to anything that they have to say, going to counseling will not be very beneficial to you.

## Attend All Recommended Sessions

Having a new baby can take a serious toll on someone, especially when it comes to those who are dealing with depression problems. Even so, it is important that you make it to all of the counseling sessions that you are scheduled for. This may seem like a great deal to worry about in addition to having to care for your child, but it is essential and you need to find some way to work this into your routine.

**Consider The Counseling Style**

Every counselor has their own way of doing things and not every method is useful for each patient. For example, there are some people offered a therapy model called Interpersonal Psychotherapy. This is when the counselor you work with is quite active during the treatment process in the hopes that they can help you find a viable solution in a limited amount of time. While this is shorter than some of the other therapy models available, it is said to be the most effective for people who suffer from postnatal depression.

**Be Open And Honest**

The only way that you will be able to find a solution to your problem is to be totally open about everything you are dealing with. From the sleepless nights to the grief and everything in between, it is essential that you discuss all of these with your counselor. Based on what you tell them, they will be able to help your sort things through, so even if it is rather difficult, you should focus all of your energy on opening up and letting your feelings show.

Counseling is one of the most popular treatments for postpartum depression. Even so, it can only be effective if you are willing to work at it. Use the advice here to help you find a great provider and glean the most benefit from the time you spend with them.

# ALTERNATIVE TREATMENT METHODS

If you are looking for something that is non-medical to treat your postpartum depression, there are options for you. Many of the side effects of pharmaceuticals and hormones make alternative treatments a more attractive choice to some people. Here are several alternative treatment methods you may want to consider.

**Acupuncture**

This is a treatment that is used to treat everything from depression to thyroid issues. Regardless of the reason behind your symptoms, acupuncture can help diminish them. While it may seem a bit nerve-wracking to imagine needles being inserted underneath the skin, they are not painful at all. Most people describe the procedure as being barely noticeable after a few treatments.

**Yoga**

Relaxing the mind and body can certainly assist you, which is where yoga comes in. This is a solid solution that has no harmful side effects and the only discomfort you will feel is trying to bend in positions that are not conducive to your body type. There are yoga classes offered in many places that are particularly for moms that are battling postnatal depression. In fact, many of these classes offer you the opportunity to bring your baby with you if you do not have a sitter.

**Reiki**

This is a Buddhist practice that involves healing in the form of laying hands on the sufferer. It may sound a bit different from what you are used to, but some people swear by it. Keep in mind that there is no proven research that shows Reiki has any positive effect on any medical conditions, yet it may be worth a shot if you have not been having any luck with any of the other methods you have tried.

## Massage Therapy

While postnatal depression is more serious than the experience of every day stress, this does not mean that massages will not be very therapeutic in this situation. Talk to your provider and give them a general idea of the stress you have been under. They can use this information to tailor your visit and provide you with a massage session that can tremendously reduce stress levels. As a result, you may notice a lower intensity in your symptoms after your sessions.

## Supplements

There are several nutritional supplements out there that can have a positive effect on the symptoms of postpartum depression. Trying one of these may be a bit safer than using pharmaceuticals, but keep in mind that some of the supplements that may have been recommended by others may not have the effect you were looking for. Popular supplement choices include vitamin B9 and S-adenosyl methionine (Sam-E).

## Essential Oils

Adding a few drops of essential oils to your bath water can help reduce some of the symptoms you have been dealing with. For example, lavender and chamomile can help with the fatigue while orange and jasmine can boost your mood and make your feel rejuvenated. It is recommended that you blend the oil with a little milk before adding them to your water. This will prevent the oil from causing any skin irritation.

There are many people who would rather from a non-medical approach to their problems before going to the nearest pharmacy and picking up a prescription. The idea is to make the choice that is best for you. If you are not sold on the idea of having medical treatments or speaking to a counselor, you may want to try one of these methods to see if you have a better experience.

# TALKING TO YOUR PARTNER

Whether you are married, engaged or currently in a relationship, your partner may have a difficult time understanding what it is you are going through. This is not as simple as willing things to be better and hoping for the best. It is important for you to help them grasp the seriousness of the situation. Try these methods if you want to have a better chance of reaching them.

## Compile Some Literature

Sometimes it is not easy to open your mouth and be direct when it comes to your feelings. As a result, it may be difficult to convey just how serious your bout with postnatal depression is. Try printing some materials that explain the situation in depth. Stay away from information that is far too technical since it may prove to be confusing. The simpler it is for your partner to understand, the better they will be when it comes to helping you through this.

## Take Them With You To Counseling

When you are dealing with postpartum depression, this is something that is felt by everyone in the household. As a result, it can take a toll on your marriage. One good way to communicate with your partner would be to do it during a therapy session. Your counselor can act as a mediator while you discuss the situation and look for ways to make it easier on both of you.

## Try To Be Understanding

Yes, you are the one that is dealing with depression, but that does not give you the right to be insensitive to the feelings of others. Just as you want them to see things from your perspective; you have to be willing to do the same. Imagine you are in their shoes and use these channeled emotions to help you better understand what they are coping with.

**Prepare For The Worst**

It is not always a wise idea to walk into a situation preparing for the worst, but that may work to your benefit in this instance. You don't want to be overly positive since this may make the blow harder if you don't receive the response that you had hoped for. While you are not being instructed to assume the worst is going to happen, you are being advised to prepare yourself mentally in order to avoid a setback.

**Answer Any Questions They May Have**

This may seem like a personal problem and it may be difficult being starkly honest with others about it, but it is absolutely necessary. You do not want to have them walk into the situation filled with doubt and wonder and walk away in the same place. Allow them to ask questions and make sure to provide them with all of the answers. It is a small concession to give someone who is willing to help you through a difficult time.

It is never easy to open your mind and reveal all of the contents with the one you love. While you may have a great relationship otherwise, this is one of those things that make people feel vulnerable. This is a hard thing to do, so conjure up the strength and try your best to be open with them.

# TAKING CARE OF YOURSELF

One thing that you may have noticed since you have been dealing with postpartum depression is the overwhelming desire to falter in caring for oneself. Things that used to be second nature to you may seem like a chore at this point. Here are some pointers you may need if you find your self-care regimen slipping.

**Get Dressed Daily**

One way to make yourself feel much better is getting dressed each and every day; even if you have nowhere to go. When you walk around the house in pajamas all day, it promotes the depressing feelings that you are fighting to overcome and defeat. No one is telling you that you need to get up and put on an evening gown or a suit, but you should make it a point to change into something other than what you wore to bed.

**Eat Regularly**

It is sometimes easy to forget to eat when you are caring for a little one and depression has started to sink in. If you are having a hard time remembering this, you should try setting an alarm. Appetite loss is a significant aspect of postpartum depression, but it is important that you eat something. Even if you have to consume meal replacement shakes, that is better than not having anything at all.

**Do Your Hair**

Ponytails are the norm for moms everywhere, but you should consider doing something a little different. Placing your hair in an updo is a bit more elegant, yet it serves the same general purpose as a ratty ponytail. You probably had much more time to do your hair before the baby arrived, but this should not stop you from taking the time to neaten your tresses.

## Stay Away From Drugs

Sometimes when things seem to be spinning out of control, people turn to drugs. This is not only a crutch that can take a toll on your physical health; it can push your emotions into even more of a tailspin than they already were. While you may get a temporary good feeling when using drugs, it will be replaced with worsened feelings once their effects wear off and you are no longer under their influence. Being high will also hinder your ability to be the parent your child needs.

## Watch Your Alcohol Intake

There is nothing wrong with having a glass of wine or two if you need to unwind, but drinking excessively can cause more harm than ever. How can you take care of your child if you are so inebriated that your actions are impaired? You do not want a small indulgence to turn into a serious drinking problem, so be mindful.

## Stay On Top Of Your Hygiene

When it feels as if life is not going your way, it can be easy to forget about things like bathing, brushing your teeth and other general hygiene tasks. This is a huge mistake since it can lead to greater problems. For example, not taking care of your teeth can result in things like plaque buildup, gingivitis and tooth loss. It may seem like a huge burden to get up each day and clean yourself up, but you must force yourself to get it done.

## Physical Fitness

It is important for everyone to have a physical fitness routine. Whether this means doing vigorous exercise at your local gym, or doing step aerobics in your den, this is necessary to keep your body fit and your heart pumping as well as it should. Allowing yourself to lie around each day doing nothing can lead to bedsores and other maladies. Even if you only get up and walk to the local market, it is a good idea for you to stay active.

Postpartum depression tends to cloud the mind and make it feel as is everything else is not as important. If you have noticed that you are not taking very good care of yourself, this is something you should definitely work on. You do not want to sit back and wait for things to work themselves out since this will allow things to become worse than they have ever been.

# CHANGING YOUR DIET

Eating well is something that everyone should be doing, yet new moms are notorious for grabbing whatever they can whenever they can. This convenience culture makes it difficult to make good eating choices. While some doctors are hesitant to say that eating better will have a direct impact on treating depression, others feel that it has a direct correlation.

If you were smaller before and you have gained weight as a result of having your baby, this can contribute to some of the negative feelings you are experiencing. This is why eating well needs to be at the top of your list of things to do. Here are several tips you should keep in mind if you are looking to change your diet for the better.

**Be Careful With Calories**

One problem many people experience when they are trying to lose weight is failing to consume enough calories. While you should most certainly not be eating as much as an NFL player, you should not be eating the same amount as a young child.

The idea is to eat at least 1,000 calories each day. If you consume less than that, it will reduce the tryptophan in the body, which is the amino acid that produces serotonin. Decreased levels of serotonin have been known to cause depression in some people.

**Reduce Your Caffeine Consumption**

Having an extra dose of caffeine is something that many new moms aim for since they have so much to get done in a limited amount of time. It can give you the temporary rush you are looking for, but the after effects make consuming this a mistake. If you must have something in your system to boost your energy levels, you should talk to your doctor about B12 supplements.

**Eat Good Carbs**

There are many foods out there that contain carbs, yet some of them are not very good dietary options. Those that have been processed lack the nutritional value found in whole grains. Instead of reaching for things like white rice, white bread and white pasta, you should reach for their brown counterparts. Eating the right carbs will create a boost in serotonin, which may lead to a boost in your overall mood.

**Add Omega-3 Fatty Acids To Your Meals**

This is one of those health tips that physicians are on the fence about it, but it could be worth a shot if there is a positive outcome. There have been studies conducted that suggest people who take omega-3 fatty acids in addition to their antidepressants show a more dramatic improvement. Foods that offer this nutrient include salmon, walnuts, flaxseed and certain brands of eggs (you will need to check the label).

**Eat Many Small Meals**

Instead of eating large meals three times a day, you should consider breaking them up into many smaller ones. Ideally, you should be eating 6-8 times per day. This will help you a great deal since you will not have to wait so long between meals, which can have a huge impact on your blood sugar levels. When this number is low, it can make the negative feelings you have experienced seem far more intense.

There is no magical diet that will give every person the results they have hoped to achieve. The key is to find an eating plan that works for you and integrate these ideas into that plan. As long as you eat better, you will feel better, so try your best to follow the advice offered here.

# FINDING A SUPPORT GROUP

Even if you are currently seeing an individual counselor, it might greatly benefit you to join a support group. Talking to others who share similar issues as you has proven to be very therapeutic. There are support groups all over the place; you just have to know where to find them. Use these pointers if you need to be nudged in the right direction.

## Ask Your Counselor

Many times there are all types of counseling sessions offering at one organization. This means that you may be able to find a support group that is held at the same location you are used to. That is an added bonus since this means that you will not have to do too much adjusting when it comes to traveling to each session. Even if there are no related groups at the organization, your counselor may be able to let you know of someplace that has this as an option.

## Attend A Few Sessions

When you are an attendee if a support group, it is important that you feel comfortable interacting with the people who are in the room with you. Since there are some areas that have an abundance of available groups, you may want to sit in a session or two in order to get a general idea of what can be expected. If you feel you will not be able to mesh with the people in any of the groups you attend, it would be best to continue searching for a group that will meet your needs.

## Consider An Online Group

If you live in an area where there are not many groups to choose from and/or the idea of trying to commute to a group is too much for you, there is the possibility of attending an online group. This is somewhat different in the sense that you will be totally anonymous, and you may miss some of the personalization and intimacy that comes with getting together with a group in person.

## Call A Helpline

There are places available for parents to call when they feel that they are overwhelmed by everything that is happening to them. These helplines can be a valuable source of information for parents who are not sure of where to turn. Providing resources is a part of the services offered by most helplines, so you should consider calling them if you are looking for a support group and you are not having any luck.

## Check Local Bulletin Boards

Whether you believe it or not, there are many support groups who post on local bulletin boards in order to gain new attendees. This is because some organizations only allow groups to continue if they have people who are genuinely interested in attending. For example, if the local community center runs a postpartum depression support group and no one shows up for most of the sessions, this is a waste of time and space that could have been spent on someone else.

You will have no idea how helpful a support group can be if you are not willing to take a chance. The best way to ensure a positive experience would be to use the advice above to find one that is a good fit for you. If you attend the wrong group, it can make things much worse instead of showing an improvement.

# CONNECTING WITH OTHER ADULTS

One underlying reason for new moms being under so much stress is the fact that there may be a lack of adult companionship. Since a baby demands so much time, it can be hard to find any for things as mundane as socializing. If you are looking for solid ways to forge connections with adults, here are some great ideas.

## Join Social Media Groups

Many people do not realize this, but several social media sites allow members to join groups. For example, Facebook has numerous groups set up for adults of different backgrounds who are willing to discuss a wide range of topics. If you allow yourself to join a few of these groups and relax getting to know like-minded people, it can help you release some of the tension that you have building up inside.

## Consider Meeting Websites

There are a few websites that people these days use to meet others who have similar interests. These meetings generally occur in public areas and they are a welcome reprieve from the hectic pace of daily life. Some of these meeting websites require a fee and/or yearly dues, but they are very useful if you are looking for a new and unique way to make friends.

## Call Your Friends

Perhaps you already have friends, but you have been isolating yourself and giving them all types of excuses when it comes to making time for them. Even if you don't have time to meet and hang out with them, you should call and try to have an adult conversation. You may not have much to say, but it will be more refreshing than changing diapers all day.

## Take A Class

Is there something that you have always wanted to learn yet you never pursued it? This is something that you might want to consider at this time. Whether you are looking to earn an advanced degree or you are looking to become a master of pottery, there are classes out there calling your name. If you are concerned about childcare, consider going to a class at a community center since many of them provide this service to parents.

## Date Your Partner

Parents often get so caught up with the excitement of a new baby that they don't take the time to stay connected with one another. Get a babysitter and spend some time together at least once or twice a month. While this is not a cure-all for postnatal depression, it can certainly boost your spirits and reduce some of the negative feelings you have been having.

## Online Forums

There are forums out there for people who fit into all type of boxes, so there is guaranteed to be one that you enjoy. This is a place where you will not have to worry about the baby (unless you want to) and you will have the chance to connect with people from all over the world. If you come across one that you don't like, do not worry, there are many more to explore.

Having adult time is essential, even after you become a parent. While postpartum depression is far more serious than having a good time and willing the bad feelings to go away, having positive experiences can make your emotional burden seem lighter and easier to bear. The next thing you will need to worry about is finding ways to reduce all of the stress you have been under.

# LEARNING TO EFFECTIVELY HANDLE STRESS

One way to deal with the overwhelming feelings of depression you are experiencing would be to avoid stress as much as possible. While it is not really likely that you will be able to eliminate it as a whole, there are several methods that can be used to reduce it tremendously. Here are some ideas you should consider the next time you feel like stress is taking a toll on you.

## Keep A Journal

If you are not a very prolific writer, this may seem like something that is not very practical, but it can really help. It is not always easy to express yourself to others, yet you may feel compelled to release all of the feelings that you have been holding inside. Keeping a journal will give you a chance to express yourself without fear of judgment or misunderstandings. You may want to consider sharing this with your counselor since it can enhance the help you are getting.

## Remember Your Are Human

This may sound strange, but it is actually quite important. One reason that many new moms have issues with depression is because they feel like they are constantly letting themselves down. You have to remember that you are human and no one out there expects you to be a superhero. There will be times where you do the wrong thing and that is okay. Don't be so hard on yourself for every little thing that goes wrong.

**Stay Away From Drugs And Alcohol**

You may feel like you are having déjà vu since this was mentioned earlier, but the repeated emphasis reflects how important it is for you to remember this. There is nothing worse than falling into a drug and/or alcohol addiction when you are a mother. Not only is this a detriment to your health, but it will impair your ability to be a quality role model for your child. Always keep in mind that this is a temporary reprieve that will lead you down a darker path in the future.

**Hand Over Some Of The Responsibility**

Every child has two parents and you need to learn to delegate some responsibilities to the other parent. This is a very common problem with stay at home moms since they are generally expected to take care of everything at home. Sure, your partner may have a very demanding job, but that is no excuse for them to act as if you are the only parent. They need to step up and take some of the burden off of you.

**Take A Breather**

When you feel like you are in over your head, take a step back and assess the situation. Even if this means that you need to place yourself in timeout, that is what needs to be done. You may not have a wealth of time that can be used for mindless activities, but taking a few minutes to calm down and regroup can make a huge difference in the way stress is handled.

Stress is one of those things that affect everyone, but those with postnatal depression have a harder time handling it than others. Use any or all of the idea here if you are trying to find a solid way to handle stressful situations when they come your way. Now to discuss talking to everyone in your life and helping them understand what is going in with you.

# TALKING TO THOSE AROUND YOU

People who have postpartum depression don't act like themselves, which means that those around them may have a hard time dealing with them. It is difficult to be there for someone through a stressful time in their lives if you are not aware that an issue actually exists. Silently suffering is unhealthy and it can permanently damage the relationships you have with family, friends and others you deal with on a regular basis. Here are a few tips that will make it easier to talk to those around you about your depression.

## Have Your Partner Help You

Sometimes it is hard to discuss painful things when it concerns you, so having your partner discuss it with others is one way to get it out in the open without you feeling more uncomfortable than you need to be. If you insist on speaking with everyone yourself, it would be best to have your partner in the room showing support. Seeing them can reassure people that your depression is a very real problem, but that you are really trying to get it under control.

## Try Family Counseling

If you have other children besides the new baby, it can be very hard for them to handle the depression you are going through. As you already know by this point, just because you are the one who is depressed, that does not mean that it does not affect the lives of those around you. Many counselors have experience dealing with postpartum as well as experience working with families, so they can guide you when you are trying to figure out how to convey your feelings in a way that would be simple for children to understand.

## Call A Meeting

There is nothing worse than having to repeat information over and over. When you are already stressed out, this threatens to make the situation even worse. Instead of going to each person individually and trying to explain everything, try calling a meeting and talking to everyone at once. If you are not very comfortable, you can break things up into a few separate gatherings. This will make it easier on your since you will not have to continuously say the same things.

## Keep Calm

Unfortunately, everyone you discuss this with may not have nice things to say. You may be told that you are exaggerating and/or the feelings you are experiencing are not valid. If this happens, assure them that what you feel is very real, you respect their opinion and you do not want to discuss this with them any longer. This may seem like something that you want to remain strong and stern about, but you have to know when to let things go. You don't need any more stress building up on top of what you are already going through.

## Don't Tell Everyone

Postpartum depression is a very personal matter, so it is not something that you want to share with everyone in your life. Your partner, family, close friends and children should probably be the only ones you discuss this with outside of a professional setting. There is a stigma that often follows people who have depression and you don't want this to damage people's perception of you. Exercise discretion when deciding who to share it with.

Talking to the people in your life about something so personal may be atypical, but it is quite necessary. You do not want to lose everyone in your life because they have no explanation for the way that you have been acting lately. Use what you have learned here to make this part of the process simpler for you.

# WORKING ON GETTING MORE SLEEP

Lack of sleep can make many people feel like they are coming apart at the seams. If you are dealing with postnatal depression, there is a chance that you have had many sleepless nights. There are a few things you can try if you are looking to get more sleep than you have been, and they are highlighted here.

## Take Supplements

There are natural supplements out there that can help you get more sleep. The best thing about these things is that they are not filled with harmful chemicals or other substances that can harm you body. One example of a supplement people use to sleep better is melatonin. While it is not a sleeping pill per se, it will help you wind down from the day and get more restful sleep.

## Take Naps With The Baby

You are probably going to have many sleepless nights until the baby has found some type of sleep routine. In the meantime, you should try going to sleep every time the baby does. Whether this means that you are going to sleep at two in the morning or three in the afternoon, take the free moment to get some rest. Many moms try to use this time to do chores, but those are less important that you being at your best, which you cannot do without any rest.

## Don't Exercise Close To Bedtime

One issue that many people have is the inability to exercise due to time constraints. Do not allow something like this to lead to exercise sessions too close to bedtime. When you get your adrenaline pumping, it will take some serious winding down to prepare for sleep. As a rule, you should not exercise any less than four hours before you are planning to head to bed.

## Turn Off The Lights

You may be accustomed to falling asleep while watching television, but this is not a good way to rest. If you are distracted by the topics on the screen, it can hinder your ability to go to sleep right away. Make sure that the room you are in is dark and you are lying there in sleep mode. This is the only way that you will be able to go to sleep faster than normal.

## Don't Get Back Up

If you are in bed and you are feeling pretty restless, it is never a good idea to get back up and try to do activities that are intended to wear you out. For example, if you are in bed and sleep is not coming to you, getting up and throwing in a load of laundry is not going to make the situation any better. Once you are in bed for the night, the only things that should get you up are bathroom urges and taking care of the baby.

## Get Sleeping Pills From Your Doctor

If you have tried everything else and there is no other way for you to get any rest, you may want to ask your doctor about sleeping pills. Since you may not be able to hear the baby in the middle of the night, this is only recommended if your partner is willing to get up with the baby in the event that you are in a deep slumber. Be very careful since some people get addicted to these and cannot sleep any other way, Also, avoid taking over the counter sleep aids unless your physician told you that it was okay.

Getting a good amount of sleep makes things much easier to deal with. It is hard to handle depression when you are running on an empty tank. It is a conundrum: You cannot sleep because you are depressed and lack of sleep is worsening your symptoms. Try a few of the tips above to see if you are able to get a little more sleep.

# FITNESS TIPS FOR NEW MOMS

If you are not feeling particularly good about the way you look, it can make it quite difficult for you to function well. While you have just had a baby and it may take a while for you to regain your former shape, people with postpartum depression generally have a much harder time handling that concept than others do. Here is advice that will help you get your body back in shape.

## Grab A Friend

Working out alone is a chore and this is what stops people from exercising as much as they probably should. Try finding a buddy that you can exercise with. Ideally, it would be someone who just had a baby as well since they will be able to relate and you will feel less awkward around them. When you have a fitness buddy, it gives you a reason to work out even when you are not in the mood - trying to avoid letting them down mean that you are less likely to skip sessions.

## Create Some Reasonable Goals

If you were 110 pounds when you first conceived and you are 250 pounds now, there is no way that you will lose the weight in two weeks. These are the type of unreasonable goals that set people up to fail. The best thing to do would be to set small goals and work your way up to larger ones. Try losing 5-10 pounds at first, and then increase the number once you notice you are getting smaller.

## Don't Be So Hard On Yourself

If you miss a day at the gym or you are not able to do as many repetitions as you would like, that is fine. You should praise yourself for how well you are doing and avoid beating yourself up when things are not going as planned. You have a baby and other life responsibilities to deal with, so sometimes fitness will have to take a backseat. You can always rework your schedule and goals to make up for the slip.

**Look For Online Support**

There are many websites out there that have health trackers that were created with new moms in mind. You are allowed to enter things like BMI, height, current weight and target weight to create a plan that will help you achieve your fitness goals. Many of them are free, so you don't have to worry about paying for anything. If you try one of these sites and you are not very happy with it, try another. It may just be that the methods employed by one site are preferable to those used by another.

**Find Small Opportunities To Integrate Fitness**

In the event that you don't have the time to get any formal exercise, you can try adding it to your schedule in other ways. For example, try walking to the store instead of taking your car. Sure, that may take a little longer, but it will give you the chance to multitask. Pull out the stroller and take your baby for a walk while doing errands. This is much easier to fit into your schedule than calisthenics.

Fitness is often forgotten once a new baby arrives and this is a huge cause for concern. As long as you are unhappy with yourself, there is no way for the symptoms of postpartum to diminish. In fact, the longer you are dealing with body issues, the longer you will probably have to deal with the emotional fallout. Next are Ten Commandments every new mom should remember.

# THE TEN NEW MOM COMMANDMENTS

Being a new mother is not an easy task and it is not second nature for some people. Motherhood is not child's play (no pun intended), but it should not become the hardest thing that you have ever had to face. As long as you always remember the ten new mom commandments things should be less complicated for you.

### #1 – Thou Shalt Not Concede

Being a new mom is not something that anyone has ever said was easy. This does not mean that you should throw in the towel just because things were not as simple as you had previously imagined.

### #2 – Thou Shalt Not Cry Too Often

Yes, there will be many times when you feel like pulling out your hair, but it is important for you to remain calm. The best thing to do would be for you to remember what you learned earlier and attempt to relax.

### #3 – Thou Shalt Not Play The Blame Game

You may have postpartum depression, but that does not mean that you should blame your baby for the way that you are feeling. This is an emotional issue that needs to be handled appropriately.

## #4 – Thou Shalt Not Be Afraid Of Asking For Help

They say no man is an island, so keep this in mind when you are going through issues. As long as you try to play hero and do everything on your own, it will only make things worse.

## #5 – Thou Shalt Prioritize Well

Sometimes there is no time to get everything done. You have to know when to throw your hands up and save some for another time. Do the things that are the most important and allow everything else to wait.

## #6 – Thou Shalt Be Honest With Yourself And Others

You are a new mom, you have postpartum depression and the world seems like a dark place right now. Admit that you are having an issue and tell others what is going on with you.

## #7 – Thou Shalt Understand This Is Normal

Every mom does not experience depression after the birth of their children, but you are certainly not the only one. The sooner you convince yourself of this, the sooner you will begin to feel better about the situation.

## #8 – Thou Shalt Make The Most Of Your Situation

Yes, you have gained weight and you have on a sweatshirt that has seen better days, but you have a bundle of joy and you are in charge of being the best possible mom. Do everything you can to make that happen.

## #9 – Thou Shalt Seek Professional Help

Some people can effectively battle postnatal depression without going to a doctor or mental health clinician, but this is not always the case. If you feel like you are in over your head doing it at home, it is time to try a new approach.

## #10 – Thou Shalt Accept The Changes

Life is all about change, and being a new mom is one great way to prove this. Instead of sitting around missing a life that you once had, focus on the one that is just getting started.

As you were told many times earlier, there are no magic tricks that will make postpartum depression disappear. This is something that will need to be worked on. By integrating these commandments into your life, your depression may become easier to handle. While some of these commandments may seem to be a bit cheeky, try to remember all of this as you are beginning your journey into motherhood.

# CONCLUSION

Depression is an illness that plagues people all over the globe, the terrible thing about it is that there are many people that fail to recognize it as a legitimate problem. If you have never experienced symptoms of depression before and you notice them directly after having a child, this is a sign that you may have postnatal depression.

Don't get all bent out of shape and start trying to convince yourself that you are not crazy. This does not mean that you are losing your mind or that there is no hope for recovery. There are many people who have suffered through this in the past and they were able to work hard to find themselves again.

Everyone has days where they wake up and they would rather pull the cover back over their head than to get up. People who are depressed have feelings like this more often than not. This doesn't automatically get you branded as a bad or lazy person. What it does mean is that you need help, whether that is personal or professional depends on the severity of what you are experiencing.

If you are able to talk to those around you and have them help you restore your emotions, that is great, but it may be necessary for you to go and see a doctor. There is a stigma surrounding this, but do not let that stop you from getting the help you need. Listen to what the doctor recommends and follow it to the letter. This will make it less likely that the depression will last for an extended time.

You may have gained weight, lost time, had a messy home, changed a billion diapers and you generally feel like you are in over your head. The good thing is that there is help available.

There were many options discussed here and it is up to you to take this information and use it to your advantage.

It is now time for you to look in the mirror, admit that you are depressed and get the help you need before it is too late. If you have watched the news in the past few years, there are a few high-profile stories where new moms have done things to harm themselves, their children and/ or their spouses. You do not want this to be your fate, and this is exactly why it is being stressed that you seek help.

Tomorrow is a new day. Get up and try all of the things you have learned here and see which of them work for you. Perhaps all you need is a bit of yoga or Reiki, maybe you need to go online in a forum to vent, or perhaps you need to make an appointment with a therapist - whatever you decide to do, make sure that you do not wait too long. All that will do is lead you to days that may be darker and you may have a harder time getting back on the right track.